Table of Contents

Contents

Introduction 5
Chapter 1: Understanding Holistic Health 10
Chapter 2: Nutrition and Diet 16
Chapter 3: Physical Health and Fitness 24
Chapter 4: Mental and Emotional Well-being 33
Chapter 5: Clean Eating, The Most High's Way 38
Chapter 6: Rest and Sleep 45
Chapter 7: Preventative Healthcare 53
Chapter 8 Detoxification and Cleansing 57
Chapter 9: Common Diseases and Disorders 64
Chapter 10: Decreasing the Sugar 77
Chapter 11 Vitamins and Minerals 82
Chapter 12 Creating a Holistic Lifestyle 90
Conclusion 94
Resources for Further Reading 96
Quick and Healthy Meal Recommendation 99
Reference Page 101

Achieving Your Best Health Holistically

Achieving Your Best Health Holistically

Lisa F. Thomas

This book is dedicated to my beautiful daughters, Antoinette L. Fairbairn and Teyanna Hicks-Oliver who have always been my rock. They are the inspiration that catapults me forward in everything that I strive to achieve. I always want to be the best example for them. Further dedication goes out to my beautiful granddaughters, Rosemary and Elisabet to whom I simply love and adore. They are my little geniuses! Additionally, my sister-friend Tammie Ross who has been my closest friend for over 30 years, my dearest friends, Cynda Alexander and Debra Williams who became an intricate part of my family over 15 years ago. Lastly, my son-n-law Steven Fairbairn, other close family members and my late mother, Essie J. Madison who recently transitioned to spiritual rest June 28, 2024.

Introduction

Holistic health is an approach to health care that considers the whole person—body, mind, spirit, and emotions—in the quest for optimal health and wellness. It emphasizes the interconnectedness of these aspects and aims to treat the individual as a whole rather than focusing solely on isolated symptoms or diseases.

Key principles of holistic health include:

1. **Integration**: Recognizing the interplay between physical, mental, emotional, and spiritual well-being, and addressing these aspects collectively in treatment and prevention.
2. **Prevention**: Emphasizing proactive measures to maintain health and prevent illness through lifestyle changes, nutrition, stress management, and other natural therapies.
3. **Individualization**: Tailoring treatment plans to the unique needs of each person, considering their specific health concerns, preferences, and circumstances.

4. **Empowerment**: Encouraging individuals to take an active role in their health care decisions, promoting self-awareness, and providing tools for self-care.
5. **Balance**: Striving for a harmonious balance among the various dimensions of health to achieve overall well-being.

Holistic health practitioners may include a wide range of modalities and treatments such as acupuncture, herbal medicine, mindfulness practices, yoga, nutritional counseling, and more. The goal is to foster a state of holistic health where individuals experience vitality, resilience, and a sense of wholeness in their lives.

A holistic approach to health is crucial for several reasons, each contributing to a comprehensive and integrated understanding of well-being:

1. **Addresses Root Causes**: Unlike traditional medicine that often focuses on symptoms, a holistic approach seeks to identify and address the root causes of health issues. By considering all aspects of a person's life—physical, mental, emotional, social, and spiritual—

holistic health practitioners can develop more effective treatment plans that lead to long-term healing and prevention.

2. **Promotes Overall Well-Being**: Holistic health emphasizes the interconnectedness of various aspects of health. By nurturing not only physical health but also mental clarity, emotional stability, social connectedness, and spiritual fulfillment, individuals can achieve a balanced and fulfilling life. This approach supports a higher quality of life and a sense of vitality.

3. **Preventative Focus**: Holistic health encourages proactive measures to prevent illness and promote wellness. Through lifestyle modifications, stress management techniques, nutritional guidance, and other preventive strategies, individuals can strengthen their immune systems, reduce the risk of chronic diseases, and enhance their overall resilience to health challenges.

4. **Personalized Care**: Each person is unique, and a holistic approach recognizes this by tailoring treatment plans to individual needs and preferences. By taking into account a person's physical health status, emotional state, lifestyle habits, and personal goals, practitioners can

offer personalized care that resonates with the individual and promotes sustainable health improvements.

5. **Empowers Individuals**: Holistic health empowers individuals to take an active role in their own health and well-being. By educating patients about their bodies, health conditions, and treatment options, and by promoting self-care practices such as mindfulness, exercise, and healthy eating, individuals gain the knowledge and skills necessary to make informed decisions and maintain optimal health over time.

6. **Enhances Patient-Practitioner Relationship**: Holistic health fosters a deeper and more collaborative relationship between patients and practitioners. By considering all dimensions of health, practitioners can better understand their patients' needs, values, and goals, leading to more effective communication, trust, and mutual respect in the therapeutic process.

7. **Integrates Different Modalities**: Holistic health encourages the integration of conventional medicine with complementary and alternative therapies (CAM), such as acupuncture, herbal medicine,

chiropractic care, and mind-body practices like yoga and meditation. This integrative approach provides a wider range of treatment options and allows for a more holistic and personalized approach to health care.

Chapter 1: Understanding Holistic Health

Holistic health is an approach to health care that emphasizes the importance of the whole person—body, mind, spirit, and emotions—in achieving wellness. It recognizes that each individual is a complex integration of these interconnected dimensions, and that optimal health cannot be achieved by focusing on one aspect alone.

The connection between mind, body, and spirit is fundamental to understanding holistic health and well-being. Here's an exploration of this interconnected relationship:

1. **Mind**: The mind encompasses cognitive functions such as thoughts, beliefs, perceptions, and emotions. It influences how we perceive and interpret the world around us, as well as how we respond to events and experiences. Mental health involves maintaining a balanced and healthy mind, which can affect physical health through mechanisms such as stress response and immune function.
2. **Body**: The body refers to the physical aspect of our being—our organs, tissues, muscles, and systems (like cardiovascular, digestive,

and nervous systems). Physical health is directly influenced by factors such as nutrition, exercise, sleep, and genetics. It plays a crucial role in our overall well-being and is often the focus of traditional medical treatments.

3. **Spirit**: The spirit encompasses our sense of meaning, purpose, and connection to something greater than ourselves. It involves our values, beliefs, and the quest for transcendence and inner peace. Spiritual health relates to finding harmony, peace, and fulfillment in life, which can profoundly impact mental and physical health.

A holistic approach to health offers numerous benefits that contribute to overall well-being and quality of life. Here are some key advantages:

1. **Comprehensive Care**: Holistic health considers the whole person—mind, body, spirit, and emotions—rather than just focusing on symptoms or isolated parts of the body. This comprehensive view allows practitioners to address underlying causes of health issues and promote overall wellness.

2. **Integration of Treatments**: Holistic health integrates a variety of therapeutic modalities, including conventional medicine, complementary therapies (such as acupuncture, chiropractic care, and herbal medicine), and mind-body practices (like yoga, meditation, and tai chi). This integration provides a broader range of treatment options tailored to individual needs and preferences.

3. **Personalized Approach**: Each person is unique, and a holistic approach emphasizes personalized care. Practitioners take into account a person's specific health concerns, lifestyle factors, emotional state, and spiritual beliefs when developing treatment plans. This individualized approach enhances the effectiveness of interventions and supports long-term health outcomes.

4. **Focus on Prevention**: Holistic health places a strong emphasis on preventive care. By promoting healthy lifestyle habits, nutrition, stress management techniques, and regular physical activity, individuals can reduce their risk of developing chronic diseases and maintain optimal health.

5. **Empowerment and Self-Care**: Holistic health empowers individuals to take an active role in their own health and well-being. Through education, guidance, and encouragement of self-care practices, such as mindfulness, relaxation techniques, and dietary adjustments, individuals gain the tools and knowledge needed to make informed decisions about their health.

6. **Enhanced Quality of Life**: By addressing all aspects of health—physical, mental, emotional, social, and spiritual—holistic health practices contribute to a higher quality of life. This approach supports not only physical health but also mental clarity, emotional resilience, and a sense of purpose and fulfillment.

7. **Support for Chronic Conditions**: For individuals living with chronic illnesses or conditions, holistic health offers complementary support alongside conventional medical treatments. Integrative therapies can help manage symptoms, improve overall health outcomes, and enhance quality of life by addressing the holistic needs of the individual.

8. **Promotion of Well-being**: Holistic health promotes a sense of well-being by fostering a harmonious balance among different aspects of health. This holistic view encourages individuals to cultivate resilience, adaptability, and a positive outlook on life, even in the face of challenges.

To my reader, below are questions that you can ask yourself and reflect upon. The questions may grant personal insight regarding your own personal health goals.

What does holistic health mean to you personally? How do you integrate holistic principles into your own life?

Have you ever tried any holistic health practices or therapies (e.g., acupuncture, yoga, meditation)? What was your experience like?

How do you think the mind-body connection influences overall health? Can you share any personal experiences or observations?

What role do you believe emotional and spiritual well-being play in maintaining good health? How do you nurture these aspects in your life?

From your perspective, what are the benefits of taking a holistic approach to health care compared to a more traditional medical approach?

How do you think preventive care fits into the holistic health paradigm? What preventive measures do you prioritize in your daily life?

Have you encountered any challenges or barriers when trying to integrate holistic health practices into your lifestyle? How did you overcome them?

Chapter 2: Nutrition and Diet

A balanced diet is essential for maintaining good health and providing the body with the necessary nutrients it needs to function optimally. Here are the basics of what constitutes a balanced diet:

1. **Variety**: Include a wide variety of foods from all food groups to ensure intake of different nutrients. This includes fruits, vegetables, whole grains, lean proteins, and healthy fats.
2. **Fruits and Vegetables**: Aim to consume a variety of colorful fruits and vegetables every day. They are rich in vitamins, minerals, antioxidants, and fiber, which are vital for overall health and disease prevention.
3. **Whole Grains**: Choose whole grains such as brown rice, quinoa, oats, whole wheat bread, and whole grain pasta over refined grains. Whole grains provide fiber, vitamins, and minerals essential for energy and digestive health.
4. **Proteins**: Include a variety of protein sources in your diet, such as lean meats (e.g., chicken, turkey), fish, eggs, legumes (e.g., beans, lentils),

nuts, seeds, and tofu. Proteins are important for building and repairing tissues, as well as for maintaining muscle mass.

5. **Healthy Fats**: Incorporate sources of healthy fats into your diet, such as avocados, nuts, seeds, olive oil, and fatty fish (e.g., salmon, trout). These fats provide essential fatty acids that support brain function, hormone production, and overall cellular health.

6. **Dairy or Dairy Alternatives**: Choose low-fat or fat-free dairy products like milk, yogurt, and cheese, or dairy alternatives fortified with calcium and vitamin D, such as almond milk or soy milk.

7. **Limit Added Sugars and Salt**: Minimize consumption of foods and beverages high in added sugars, such as sugary drinks, candies, and desserts. Similarly, reduce intake of foods high in sodium (salt), such as processed and packaged foods.

8. **Stay Hydrated**: Drink plenty of water throughout the day. Water helps regulate body temperature, aids in digestion, and supports overall bodily functions.

9. **Moderation and Portion Control**: Pay attention to portion sizes and practice moderation, even with healthy foods. Eating balanced meals

and snacks throughout the day can help maintain energy levels and prevent overeating.

10. **Consider Individual Needs**: Factors such as age, gender, activity level, and health status can influence dietary needs. Consult with a registered dietitian or healthcare provider for personalized recommendations.

By following these basic principles of a balanced diet, you can ensure that your body receives the nutrients it needs for optimal health, energy, and well-being.

Whole foods, such as fruits, vegetables, whole grains, lean proteins, and healthy fats, provide essential nutrients like vitamins, minerals, antioxidants, and fiber that are vital for overall health. Unlike processed foods, which often contain added sugars, unhealthy fats, and preservatives, whole foods retain their natural integrity and nutritional value. Consuming a diet rich in whole foods supports better digestion, helps manage weight, reduces the risk of chronic diseases like heart disease, diabetes, and certain cancers, and promotes overall longevity and vitality. Therefore, prioritizing whole foods in your diet can contribute significantly to your health and well-being by providing the body with the necessary nutrients it needs to function optimally.

Nutritional Healing: Nutritional healing emphasizes the idea that food is medicine, capable of supporting the body's natural healing processes and preventing illness. It involves consuming a balanced diet rich in nutrients to optimize overall health and well-being. Key principles include:

1. **Nutrient Density**: Choosing foods that are rich in essential nutrients such as vitamins, minerals, antioxidants, and phytochemicals.
2. **Whole Foods**: Prioritizing whole, unprocessed foods over refined and processed options to retain their nutritional integrity and health benefits.
3. **Balanced Diet**: Ensuring a balanced intake of carbohydrates, proteins, fats, and fiber, tailored to individual needs and health goals.
4. **Preventive Care**: Using nutrition to prevent chronic diseases by promoting a healthy lifestyle, including regular physical activity and stress management.

5. **Personalization**: Recognizing individual differences in nutritional needs and preferences, and customizing dietary recommendations accordingly.

Superfoods: Superfoods are nutrient-dense foods that are particularly rich in vitamins, minerals, antioxidants, and other beneficial compounds. They are believed to offer exceptional health benefits beyond basic nutrition. Common examples include:

- **Berries**: Blueberries, strawberries, and raspberries are packed with antioxidants that help protect cells from damage and support overall health.
- **Leafy Greens**: Kale, spinach, and Swiss chard are high in vitamins A, C, K, and minerals like iron and calcium, supporting immune function and bone health.
- **Nuts and Seeds**: Almonds, walnuts, chia seeds, and flax seeds are rich in healthy fats, fiber, and protein, promoting heart health and satiety.

- **Fatty Fish**: Salmon, sardines, and mackerel are excellent sources of omega-3 fatty acids, which support brain function, heart health, and inflammation reduction.
- **Whole Grains**: Quinoa, oats, and brown rice provide complex carbohydrates, fiber, and essential nutrients, supporting energy levels and digestive health.

Meal Planning and Preparation tips

Meal planning and preparation can simplify healthy eating and save time. Here are some examples of tips for effective meal planning and preparation:

1. Set Aside Time for Planning: Dedicate a specific day each week to plan your meals. Consider your schedule, preferences, and nutritional needs when selecting recipes.

2. Create a Grocery List: Based on your meal plan, make a detailed grocery list. This helps streamline shopping and ensures you have all the ingredients you need.

3. Focus on Balanced Meals: Include a variety of foods from different food groups: fruits, vegetables, whole grains, lean proteins, and healthy fats.

4. Batch Cooking: Prepare large batches of staple foods like grains, proteins (e.g., chicken, beans), and vegetables that can be used in multiple meals throughout the week.

5. Prep Ingredients Ahead of Time: Wash, chop, and portion fruits, vegetables, and other ingredients in advance. Store them in containers or bags for quick and easy access during meal preparation.

6. Use Time-Saving Appliances: Utilize kitchen tools like slow cookers, instant pots, and air fryers to simplify cooking and reduce hands-on time.

7. Choose Quick and Easy Recipes: Look for recipes that require minimal preparation and cooking time, such as stir-fries, salads, one-pot meals, or sheet pan dinners.

8. Plan for Leftovers: Cook extra portions intentionally to have leftovers for future meals. This can save time and reduce food waste.

9. Pack Meals in Advance: Prepare and pack lunches or snacks the night before to grab-and-go during busy days.

10. Stay Flexible: Allow for flexibility in your meal plan to accommodate changes in schedule or unexpected events. Have backup options like frozen meals or pantry staples.

11. Experiment with Meal Prep Containers: Invest in reusable containers suitable for storing and reheating meals. Divide meals into individual portions for easy grab-and-go options.

12. Include Variety: Incorporate different flavors, textures, and cuisines into your meal plan to keep meals interesting and enjoyable.

By incorporating these meal planning and preparation tips into your routine, you can streamline the cooking process, make healthier choices, and save time during busy weekdays. It also helps foster a habit of mindful eating and supports overall well-being through balanced nutrition.

Chapter 3: Physical Health and Fitness

Regular exercise offers numerous benefits for physical, mental, and emotional well-being:

- **Physical Health**: Improves cardiovascular health, strengthens muscles and bones, enhances flexibility and endurance, and helps manage weight.
- **Mental Health**: Reduces stress, anxiety, and depression by releasing endorphins (feel-good hormones) and promoting better sleep.
- **Longevity**: Reduces the risk of chronic diseases such as heart disease, diabetes, and certain cancers.
- **Energy Levels**: Increases energy and stamina throughout the day.

Different Types of Physical Activities

- **Cardiovascular Exercise**: Activities like walking, running, cycling, swimming, and dancing that elevate heart rate and improve cardiovascular fitness.

- **Strength Training**: Involves lifting weights, using resistance bands, or bodyweight exercises to build muscle strength, improve metabolism, and enhance bone density.
- **Flexibility and Balance**: Practices such as yoga, Pilates, and stretching exercises that improve flexibility, balance, and posture.
- **Functional Training**: Incorporates movements that mimic everyday activities to improve overall fitness and mobility.

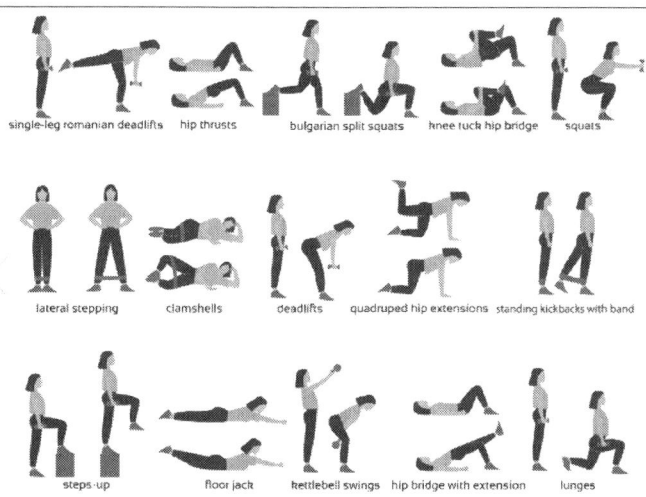

Creating a Sustainable Fitness Routine

- **Set Realistic Goals**: Establish achievable fitness goals based on your current fitness level and personal preferences.

- **Plan Variety**: Incorporate a mix of cardio, strength training, flexibility, and balance exercises to target different aspects of fitness.
- **Schedule Regular Workouts**: Dedicate specific times in your weekly schedule for exercise sessions, treating them like appointments that cannot be missed.
- **Start Gradually**: Begin with manageable intensity and duration, gradually increasing as your fitness improves.
- **Listen to Your Body**: Pay attention to how your body feels during and after exercise to prevent injury and overtraining.
- **Track Progress**: Monitor your progress by keeping a workout journal or using fitness apps to stay motivated and celebrate achievements.

Tips for Staying Motivated

- **Find Your Why**: Identify your reasons for wanting to exercise, whether it's improving health, reducing stress, or achieving specific fitness goals.
- **Mix It Up**: Keep workouts interesting by trying new activities, classes, or outdoor exercises.

- **Buddy Up**: Exercise with a friend, family member, or join group fitness classes for accountability and social support.
- **Reward Yourself**: Treat yourself to non-food rewards when you achieve milestones or consistently stick to your fitness routine.
- **Visualize Success**: Imagine yourself achieving your fitness goals and visualize the benefits of regular exercise in your daily life.
- **Stay Positive**: Focus on the positive changes exercise brings to your health and well-being, rather than solely on physical appearance.

By incorporating these elements into your fitness routine, you can create a sustainable approach to exercise that enhances overall health, boosts mood, and increases energy levels for a healthier lifestyle.

Example of exercises to promote physical fitness

Cardiovascular Endurance:

1. **Running/Jogging:**

- **Description:** Running or jogging at a moderate to vigorous pace.
- **Benefits:** Improves cardiovascular health, enhances stamina, and burns calories.

2. **Cycling:**
    - **Description:** Riding a bicycle indoors (stationary bike) or outdoors.
    - **Benefits:** Strengthens leg muscles, improves heart health, and is low-impact.

3. **Jump Rope:**
    - **Description:** Skipping rope continuously at a moderate pace.
    - **Benefits:** Increases heart rate, improves coordination, and enhances agility.

Strength Training:

1. **Bodyweight Exercises:**
    - **Push-Ups:**

- **Description:** Lowering and raising the body using arm strength while keeping the body straight.
- **Benefits:** Builds upper body and core strength.
  - **Squats:**
    - **Description:** Lowering the body by bending at the knees and hips, then returning to a standing position.
    - **Benefits:** Strengthens leg muscles (quadriceps, hamstrings, glutes) and improves lower body mobility.

2. **Resistance Band Exercises:**
   - **Banded Rows:**
     - **Description:** Holding resistance bands with both hands, pulling elbows back and squeezing shoulder blades together.
     - **Benefits:** Strengthens upper back and improves posture.
   - **Banded Leg Press:**
     - **Description:** Securing a resistance band around feet and pushing legs outward against resistance.

- **Benefits:** Targets inner thigh muscles (adductors) and improves hip stability.

Flexibility and Balance:

1. **Yoga:**
   - **Downward Facing Dog:**
     - **Description:** Forming an inverted V shape with the body, hands and feet on the ground.
     - **Benefits:** Stretches hamstrings, calves, and shoulders, improves spinal flexibility, and enhances overall body awareness.

2. **Pilates:**
   - **Single Leg Circle:**
     - **Description:** Lying on back with one leg extended, circling the leg in the air while maintaining core engagement.
     - **Benefits:** Improves hip mobility, strengthens core muscles, and enhances balance.

Core Strength:

1. **Plank:**
   - **Description:** Holding a push-up position with the body straight and supported on forearms and toes.
   - **Benefits:** Strengthens core muscles (abdominals, obliques, lower back) and improves overall stability.
2. **Russian Twists:**
   - **Description:** Sitting on the floor with knees bent, rotating torso from side to side while holding a weight or medicine ball.
   - **Benefits:** Targets oblique muscles (side abdominals), improves rotational strength, and enhances core stability.

Sample Workout Routine:

- **Warm-Up:** 5-10 minutes of light cardio (e.g., jogging in place, jumping jacks).
- **Strength Training (Circuit):** Perform each exercise for 1 minute, with 15-30 seconds of rest between exercises:
  - Push-Ups

- Squats
- Banded Rows
- Banded Leg Press

- **Cardiovascular Endurance:** Choose one activity and perform for 15-20 minutes (e.g., running, cycling).
- **Flexibility and Balance:** Finish with 10-15 minutes of yoga or Pilates focusing on stretching and balance exercises.
- **Cool Down:** Stretch major muscle groups (hamstrings, quadriceps, and calves) for 5-10 minutes to promote flexibility and reduce muscle soreness.

This sample workout routine incorporates exercises that target different aspects of physical fitness, providing a well-rounded approach to improving overall health and well-being. Adjust the intensity and duration based on individual fitness levels and goals.

Chapter 4: Mental and Emotional Well-being

Managing stress and anxiety involves adopting strategies to reduce their impact on mental and physical well-being:

1. **Identifying Triggers**: Recognize stressors and anxiety triggers to develop coping strategies.
2. **Healthy Lifestyle**: Maintain a balanced diet, regular exercise, and adequate sleep to support overall resilience.
3. **Stress Reduction Techniques**: Practice relaxation techniques such as deep breathing, meditation, yoga, or progressive muscle relaxation.
4. **Time Management**: Organize tasks, prioritize responsibilities, and delegate when possible to reduce feelings of overwhelm.
5. **Seeking Support**: Connect with friends, family, or a counselor for emotional support and perspective.
6. **Limiting Stimulants**: Reduce consumption of caffeine, alcohol, and nicotine, which can exacerbate anxiety symptoms.

Positive thinking and mindfulness promote mental well-being and resilience:

1. **Optimism and Gratitude**: Cultivate a positive outlook by focusing on strengths, achievements, and gratitude.
2. **Mindfulness Practices**: Practice mindfulness to observe thoughts and emotions without judgment, reducing stress and anxiety.
3. **Affirmations**: Use positive affirmations to challenge negative self-talk and reinforce confidence and self-esteem.
4. **Visualization**: Visualize success and positive outcomes to enhance motivation and reduce stress.
5. **Stress Reduction**: Mindfulness-based stress reduction (MBSR) techniques help manage stress through mindful awareness and meditation.
6. **Mindful Breathing**: Utilize deep breathing exercises to promote relaxation and focus during stressful situations.

Emotional resilience refers to the ability to adapt and bounce back from adversity, trauma, or stress. It involves the capacity to remain flexible in the face of difficult situations, to maintain a balanced perspective, and to cope effectively with life's challenges. Emotional resilience does not mean avoiding stress or hardships, but rather developing skills and behaviors that enable individuals to navigate through them in a healthy and constructive manner.

Learning from life's setbacks is a crucial aspect of personal growth and resilience. Setbacks provide opportunities to strengthen resilience by facing and overcoming challenges. Each experience of resilience helps build emotional strength and adaptability for future adversities. Setbacks encourage introspection and self-awareness. Reflecting on what went wrong, how it affected you, and what you can learn from it enhances personal insight and growth. It highlights areas where you excel and areas that may need improvement. Understanding your strengths can reinforce confidence, while recognizing weaknesses allows for targeted personal development.

Below are some questions to ask yourself to see how you handle life setbacks, coping skills and contributions to your personal growth. Think about your recent setback and answer the following questions:

Looking back, what strategies or coping mechanisms helped you navigate through this setback?

Did you seek support from others during this challenging period? How did they assist you?

What did you learn about yourself through overcoming this setback?

Have you experienced other setbacks in your life, and how did you handle them differently?

In what ways did this setback contribute to your personal growth or development?

Did this experience change your priorities, goals, or perspective on life?

Have you discovered any strengths or qualities within yourself that you didn't realize you had before facing this challenge?

How do you think you have become a stronger or more resilient person as a result of overcoming this setback?

What specific lessons did you learn from this setback that you carry with you today?

How has this experience influenced the way you approach future challenges or difficult situations?

What advice would you give to someone else who is currently facing a setback or adversity in their life?

Looking back, is there anything you would have done differently in handling this setback?

Chapter 5: Clean Eating, The Most High's Way

What does the Holy Bible say about your health and wellness?

Body as a Temple: "Do you not know that your bodies are temples of the Holy Spirit, who is in you, whom you have received from God? You are not your own; you were bought at a price. Therefore, honor God with your bodies." - 1 Corinthians 6:19-20 (NIV)

Moderation: "So, whether you eat or drink, or whatever you do, do everything for the glory of God." - 1 Corinthians 10:31 (NIV)

Healing and Compassion: Jesus often healed the sick and demonstrated compassion for those suffering from physical and spiritual ailments (e.g., Matthew 9:35).

Health and Healing: "He said, 'If you will heed the Lord your God diligently, doing what is upright in His sight, giving ear to His commandments and keeping all His laws, then I will not bring upon you any of the diseases that I brought upon the Egyptians, for I the Lord am your healer.'" - Exodus 15:26 (NIV)

Dietary Laws: Kosher dietary laws (kashrut) emphasize clean and healthy eating practices to maintain physical and spiritual purity.

Examples of the dietary laws found in Deuteronomy

Clean (Permissible) Foods:

1. **Land Animals**:
    - Cattle (e.g., cows, bulls)
    - Sheep/Lamb
    - Goats
    - Deer
    - Antelope
    - Gazelle
    - Roebuck

2. **Birds**:
    - Chicken
    - Turkey
    - Duck
    - Quail

- Pigeon (dove)
- Geese (some interpretations include)

3. **Fish**:
   - Fish with fins and scales (e.g., salmon, tuna, cod)
   - Perch
   - Sole
   - Haddock
   - Trout
   - Mackerel

4. **Insects** (rarely consumed, but mentioned):
   - Locusts (some interpretations)

5. **Reptiles** (rarely consumed, but mentioned):
   - Certain species of locust, such as locusts

Example Recipes for clean eating

Grilled Herb-Crusted Chicken

Ingredients:

- 4 boneless, skinless chicken breasts
- 2 tablespoons olive oil
- 2 cloves garlic, minced
- 1 teaspoon dried thyme
- 1 teaspoon dried rosemary
- 1 teaspoon dried oregano
- Salt and pepper to taste

Instructions:

1. In a small bowl, mix together olive oil, minced garlic, thyme, rosemary, oregano, salt, and pepper.
2. Rub the herb mixture evenly over the chicken breasts, covering both sides.
3. Preheat the grill to medium-high heat. Grill chicken for 6-7 minutes per side, or until cooked through and no longer pink in the center.
4. Remove from the grill and let rest for a few minutes before serving.

Serve the grilled herb-crusted chicken with a side of steamed vegetables or a fresh green salad for a balanced meal.

Baked Salmon with Lemon and Dill

Ingredients:

- 4 salmon filets (about 6 ounces each), skin-on
- 2 tablespoons olive oil
- 1 lemon, thinly sliced
- 2 tablespoons fresh dill, chopped
- Salt and pepper to taste

Instructions:

1. Preheat the oven to 400°F (200°C). Line a baking sheet with parchment paper.
2. Place the salmon filets on the baking sheet, skin-side down. Drizzle olive oil over the salmon and season with salt and pepper.
3. Arrange lemon slices on top of the salmon filets and sprinkle with chopped dill.

4. Bake in the preheated oven for 12-15 minutes, or until salmon flakes easily with a fork and is cooked to your desired doneness.
5. Serve the baked salmon with roasted vegetables or a quinoa salad for a nutritious meal.

Lentil and Vegetable Stew

Ingredients:

- 1 cup green or brown lentils, rinsed and drained
- 2 carrots, diced
- 2 celery stalks, diced
- 1 onion, diced
- 3 cloves garlic, minced
- 1 can (14 ounces) diced tomatoes
- 4 cups vegetable broth
- 1 teaspoon dried thyme
- 1 teaspoon dried rosemary
- Salt and pepper to taste

Instructions:

1. In a large pot, heat olive oil over medium heat. Add diced onion, carrots, and celery. Cook until vegetables are softened, about 5-7 minutes.
2. Add minced garlic, dried thyme, and dried rosemary. Cook for another minute until fragrant.
3. Stir in rinsed lentils, diced tomatoes (with juices), and vegetable broth. Season with salt and pepper.
4. Bring the stew to a boil, then reduce heat to low. Cover and simmer for 25-30 minutes, or until lentils are tender.
5. Adjust seasoning if needed and serve the lentil and vegetable stew hot, garnished with fresh herbs if desired.

These recipes incorporate clean foods such as chicken, salmon, vegetables, and legumes, adhering to the dietary guidelines found in Deuteronomy. They are nutritious, flavorful, and suitable for those following dietary laws that emphasize clean eating practices.

Chapter 6: Rest and Sleep

Quality sleep is essential for overall health and well-being, impacting various aspects of physical and mental functioning:

1. Physical Health: Promotes immune function, supports cardiovascular health, and aids in proper hormone regulation.
2. Mental Health: Enhances cognitive function, memory consolidation, and mood regulation.
3. Emotional Regulation: Helps manage stress, reduces irritability, and promotes emotional resilience.
4. Physical Recovery: Facilitates muscle repair, growth, and recovery after physical activity.
5. Metabolic Health: Regulates appetite hormones and supports healthy metabolism.

Tips for Better Sleep Hygiene

1. Consistent Sleep Schedule: Go to bed and wake up at the same time every day, even on weekends.

2. Create a Relaxing Bedtime Routine: Wind down before bed with calming activities like reading or taking a warm bath.
3. Optimize Sleep Environment: Keep your bedroom dark, quiet, and at a comfortable temperature.
4. Limit Screen Time: Avoid screens (phones, tablets, computers) at least an hour before bedtime to reduce exposure to blue light.
5. Watch Your Diet: Avoid heavy meals, caffeine, and alcohol close to bedtime.
6. Regular Exercise: Engage in regular physical activity, but avoid vigorous exercise too close to bedtime.
7. Manage Stress: Practice relaxation techniques such as deep breathing or meditation to calm the mind before sleep.

Understanding Sleep Cycles and Their Impact on Health

1. Sleep Stages: Include REM (Rapid Eye Movement) and Non-REM stages that cycle throughout the night.
2. Role in Memory Consolidation: REM sleep supports learning and memory consolidation processes.

3. Physical Restoration: Non-REM sleep is crucial for physical recovery and growth.
4. Hormonal Regulation: Sleep cycles help regulate hormones involved in appetite, stress response, and growth.

Restorative Practices for Relaxation

1. Mindfulness Meditation: Promotes relaxation and reduces stress.
2. Progressive Muscle Relaxation: Tensing and relaxing muscle groups to release tension.
3. Yoga and Stretching: Improves flexibility and promotes relaxation through gentle movements.
4. Breathing Exercises: Deep breathing techniques to calm the mind and body.
5. Warm Bath or Shower: Helps relax muscles and signals to the body that it's time to wind down.

By prioritizing quality sleep and incorporating good sleep hygiene practices, individuals can optimize their physical, mental, and emotional well-being.

Understanding sleep cycles and engaging in restorative practices further supports relaxation and promotes overall health.

What is the recommended amount of sleep?

The amount of sleep and rest needed varies based on age, individual factors, and overall health. Here are general guidelines for different age groups:

Infants (0-12 months):

- **Recommended Sleep**: 14-17 hours per day, including naps.
- **Sleep Patterns**: Infants typically sleep in short cycles throughout the day and night.

Toddlers (1-2 years):

- **Recommended Sleep**: 11-14 hours per day, including naps.
- **Sleep Patterns**: Transitioning to fewer naps and more consolidated nighttime sleep.

Preschoolers (3-5 years):

- **Recommended Sleep**: 10-13 hours per day.

- **Sleep Patterns**: Naps may decrease or stop; regular nighttime sleep is important.

School-Age Children (6-12 years):

- **Recommended Sleep**: 9-12 hours per day.
- **Sleep Patterns**: Establishing consistent bedtime routines and sleep schedules.

Teenagers (13-18 years):

- **Recommended Sleep**: 8-10 hours per day.
- **Sleep Patterns**: Biological changes may affect sleep patterns; maintaining a regular sleep schedule is important.

Adults (18-64 years):

- **Recommended Sleep**: 7-9 hours per day.
- **Sleep Patterns**: Quality of sleep becomes crucial; establishing good sleep hygiene is beneficial.

Older Adults (65+ years):

- **Recommended Sleep**: 7-8 hours per day.
- **Sleep Patterns**: Sleep patterns may change with age; maintaining healthy sleep habits is important for overall health.

Rest Recommendations:

- **Rest and Relaxation**: In addition to nighttime sleep, incorporating periods of rest and relaxation during the day can help recharge energy levels and reduce stress.
- **Napping**: Short naps (20-30 minutes) can be beneficial for boosting alertness and performance during the day, especially if nighttime sleep is inadequate.

Individual Variations:

- **Listen to Your Body**: Individual sleep needs can vary; pay attention to how you feel during the day to determine if you're getting enough sleep.

- **Quality of Sleep**: It's not just about the quantity but also the quality of sleep; prioritize creating a conducive sleep environment and practicing good sleep hygiene.

These recommendations provide a general framework for understanding sleep needs across different age groups. Adjustments may be necessary based on individual health conditions, lifestyle factors, and personal preferences.

Sleep and your immune system

Sleep plays a crucial role in promoting a healthy immune system through various mechanisms. During sleep, the body produces cytokines, proteins that help regulate the immune response. These cytokines are crucial in promoting sleep and combating infections. Adequate sleep helps regulate inflammation levels in the body. Chronic inflammation is linked to various health conditions, including heart disease, diabetes, and autoimmune disorders.

Sleep is essential for the production of antibodies that target and neutralize bacteria and viruses. This process strengthens the body's immune defense against infections. Sleep allows for cellular repair and regeneration, which is vital for maintaining immune system function. This process supports the body's ability to recover from daily wear and tear and prepares it to fight off pathogens.

Quality sleep helps regulate stress hormones like cortisol. Chronic stress can weaken the immune system, making it less effective in responding to pathogens. Sleep plays a role in memory consolidation and learning processes. These cognitive functions indirectly support immune health by promoting overall well-being and stress management. Consistent and sufficient sleep contributes to overall health maintenance, reducing the risk of chronic illnesses that can compromise immune function over time.

Chapter 7: Preventive Healthcare

Regular check-ups and screenings are crucial for maintaining overall health and detecting potential health issues early. Routine check-ups allow healthcare providers to identify health problems in their early stages when they may be more easily treatable. Screenings such as blood pressure checks, cholesterol tests, and cancer screenings help monitor health status and identify risk factors.

Regular visits to healthcare providers or holistic practitioners enable monitoring of chronic conditions and adjustment of treatment plans as needed. Check-ups provide opportunities for healthcare professionals to educate patients about healthy lifestyle choices, disease prevention, and early warning signs.

Incorporating natural remedies and preventive measures into daily routines can support overall health and well-being. Eating a balanced diet rich in fruits, vegetables, whole grains, and lean proteins supports immune function and overall health. Regular exercise improves cardiovascular health, strengthens muscles and bones, and reduces the risk of chronic diseases.

Practices such as meditation, strength exercises, and deep breathing techniques help reduce stress levels and promote mental well-being. Establishing a consistent sleep schedule and creating a conducive sleep environment supports immune function and overall health. Drinking an adequate amount of water daily promotes proper bodily functions and overall health.

The importance of drinking adequate water

Drinking an adequate amount of water is crucial for maintaining overall health and well-being due to several important reasons:

1. **Hydration**: Water is essential for proper hydration of the body. It helps regulate body temperature, transport nutrients and oxygen to cells, and remove waste products.
2. **Healthy Skin**: Adequate hydration supports skin health by maintaining elasticity, reducing dryness, and promoting a healthy glow. Dehydration can lead to dry, flaky skin and exacerbate skin conditions like eczema.

3. **Digestive Health**: Water aids in digestion and prevents constipation by keeping the digestive system functioning smoothly. It helps dissolve nutrients and ensures their proper absorption.

4. **Kidney Function**: Water plays a key role in kidney function by helping to flush out waste products and toxins through urine. Dehydration can strain the kidneys and contribute to the formation of kidney stones.

5. **Joint Lubrication**: Proper hydration keeps joints lubricated and cushions them against impact. This can help reduce joint pain and improve joint function, especially important for those with arthritis or joint problems.

6. **Energy Levels**: Staying hydrated supports energy levels and cognitive function. Dehydration can lead to feelings of fatigue, difficulty concentrating, and reduced physical performance.

7. **Weight Management**: Drinking water before meals can help reduce calorie intake and support weight loss efforts. It promotes a feeling of fullness, which may prevent overeating.

8. **Detoxification**: Water is essential for the body's natural detoxification processes, helping to flush out toxins and waste products from various organs and tissues.

Tips for Ensuring Adequate Hydration:

- **Drink throughout the Day**: Aim to drink water consistently throughout the day rather than consuming large amounts at once.
- **Monitor Urine Color**: Check urine color; pale yellow indicates adequate hydration, while darker colors may indicate dehydration.
- **Consider Activity Levels**: Increase water intake during hot weather or when engaging in physical activity to replenish fluids lost through sweating.
- **Incorporate Hydrating Foods**: Eat fruits and vegetables with high water content, such as watermelon, cucumber, and oranges.

By prioritizing regular water intake, individuals can support their overall health, enhance bodily functions, and maintain optimal well-being.

Chapter 8: Detoxification and Cleansing

Body detoxification and cleansing refer to practices or processes aimed at removing toxins and impurities from the body. The concept revolves around the idea that accumulated toxins from environmental pollutants, processed foods, and other sources can build up in the body over time, potentially leading to health problems.

The body has its own natural detoxification processes primarily managed by the liver, kidneys, lungs, and skin. These organs work to filter and eliminate toxins through urine, feces, sweat, and exhalation. Some detox approaches involve dietary changes or fasting to purportedly cleanse the body. These may include consuming specific foods, juices, or herbal supplements believed to support detoxification.

Drinking plenty of water and staying hydrated is often emphasized in detox practices to support kidney function and flush out toxins. Regular physical activity can aid in detoxification by increasing circulation and promoting sweat, which helps eliminate toxins through the skin.

Colon Cleanses: These procedures involve flushing the colon with water or other solutions to remove waste and toxins. However, they are controversial and not supported by scientific evidence for routine use.

Dietary Changes: Some cleansing protocols focus on eliminating processed foods, sugars, caffeine, and alcohol, and increasing intake of whole foods like fruits, vegetables, and fiber-rich grains.

Herbal Supplements: Certain herbs and supplements are marketed for their purported detoxifying properties. Examples include milk thistle for liver health or dandelion root for kidney function.

Herbs to assist with detoxifying the body

Milk Thistle:

- **Properties**: Known for its antioxidant and anti-inflammatory properties. It is primarily used to support liver health and may aid in detoxification by enhancing liver function.
- **Form**: Often taken as a supplement in capsule or liquid extract form.

Dandelion:

- **Properties**: Acts as a diuretic and supports kidney function by increasing urine production, which may help eliminate toxins from the body.
- **Form**: Leaves and roots can be consumed in tea or as a supplement.

Burdock Root:

- **Properties**: Has diuretic properties and is believed to support liver function. It is used in traditional medicine for detoxification and purifying blood.
- **Form**: Available as a supplement or in tea form.

Ginger:

- **Properties**: Known for its anti-inflammatory and digestive properties. Ginger may support detoxification by improving digestion and promoting gastrointestinal health.
- **Form**: Used fresh in cooking, as a tea, or in supplement form.

Turmeric:

- **Properties**: Contains curcumin, a compound with antioxidant and anti-inflammatory properties. Turmeric may support detoxification by enhancing liver function and reducing inflammation.
- **Form**: Often used in cooking (as a spice) or taken as a supplement.

Nettle:

- **Properties**: Acts as a diuretic and promotes detoxification by increasing urine flow and supporting kidney function.
- **Form**: Leaves can be consumed in tea or as a supplement.

Cilantro:

- **Properties**: Known for its antioxidant properties. Cilantro may help in detoxification by binding to heavy metals and facilitating their elimination from the body.
- **Form**: Used fresh in cooking or as a supplement.

Considerations:

- **Consultation**: It's important to consult with a healthcare provider or a qualified herbalist before using herbs for detoxification, especially if you have underlying health conditions or are taking medications.
- **Safety**: Some herbs may interact with medications or have side effects. Use caution and follow recommended dosages.
- **Effectiveness**: Scientific evidence supporting the effectiveness of these herbs specifically for detoxification is limited. They are often used in combination with other lifestyle changes for holistic health benefits.

Incorporating these herbs into your diet or supplement regimen should be done cautiously and as part of a balanced approach to health and well-being.

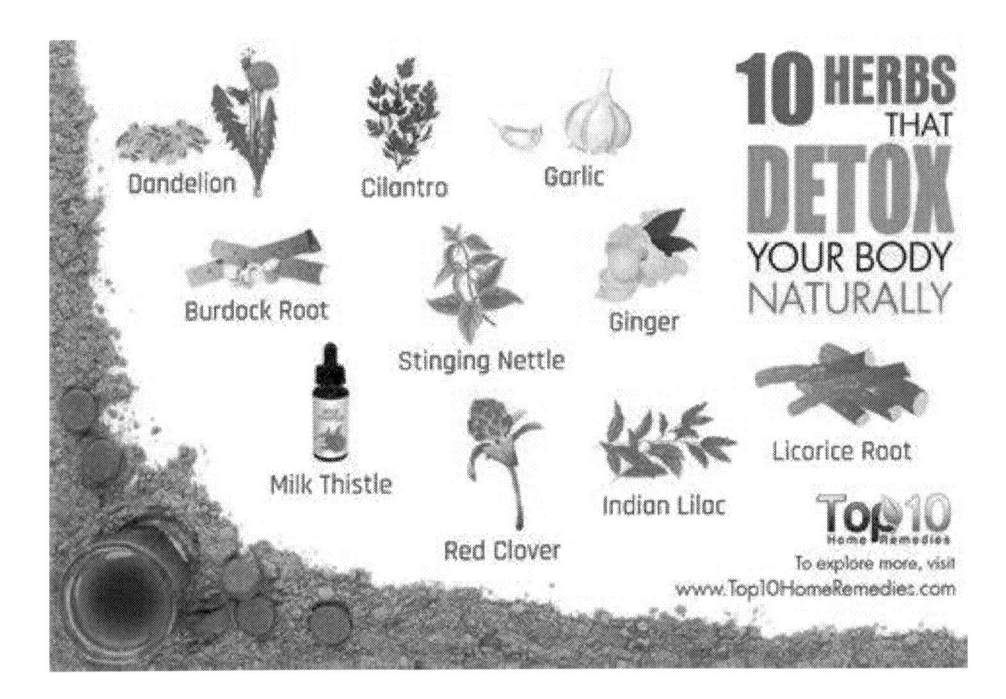

When should you detox?

The decision to engage in a detoxification regimen should be approached with caution and ideally under the guidance of a healthcare provider. Here are some considerations for when detoxification might be considered:

- **After Periods of Unhealthy Habits**: If you've had a period of unhealthy eating, excessive alcohol consumption, or exposure to environmental toxins, a detox regimen may help reset and support your body's natural detoxification processes.

- **Feeling Fatigued or Sluggish**: If you're experiencing symptoms like fatigue, bloating, or skin issues that may be related to toxin buildup, a detox program could be considered to support your body's natural cleansing mechanisms.

- **Before Starting a Healthier Lifestyle**: Some people choose to start a new health regimen, such as adopting a healthier diet or exercise routine, with a detox to kick-start the process and enhance overall results.

- **As Part of a Seasonal Cleanse**: Seasonal changes, such as transitioning from winter to spring, are often associated with detoxification practices in traditional medicine systems.

- **Medical Advice**: If you have specific health conditions related to toxin exposure or impaired detoxification pathways, your healthcare provider may recommend a detox program tailored to your needs.

Chapter 9: Common diseases and disorders

There are several common diseases and disorders where holistic approaches can complement conventional medical treatments. Holistic methods emphasize treating the whole person—mind, body, and spirit—while addressing underlying causes and promoting overall well-being. Here are some examples of conditions and herbs to consider where holistic practices may be beneficial:

Chronic Pain: Holistic approaches such as acupuncture, yoga, and mindfulness-based stress reduction (MBSR) can help manage chronic pain conditions like arthritis, fibromyalgia, and lower back pain.

Turmeric:

- **Active Compound**: Curcumin, known for its anti-inflammatory properties.
- **Uses**: Often used to reduce inflammation and pain associated with conditions like arthritis. It can be taken as a supplement or used in cooking.

Ginger:

- **Active Compounds**: Gingerol and zingerone, which have anti-inflammatory and pain-relieving properties.
- **Uses**: Used to alleviate muscle pain, arthritis pain, and migraines. Ginger can be consumed fresh, as a tea, or in supplement form.

Devil's Claw:

- **Active Compounds**: Harpagoside, known for its anti-inflammatory effects.
- **Uses**: Traditionally used to relieve joint pain and back pain. Available in supplement form.

White Willow Bark:

- **Active Compound**: Salicin, which is similar to aspirin and has anti-inflammatory and analgesic properties.
- **Uses**: Used for centuries to relieve pain and inflammation, particularly for conditions like osteoarthritis. It can be brewed as a tea or taken in supplement form.

Boswellia:

- **Active Compounds**: Boswellic acids, known for their anti-inflammatory effects.
- **Uses**: Used to reduce inflammation and pain in conditions such as osteoarthritis and rheumatoid arthritis. Available as a supplement.

Capsaicin:

- **Active Compound**: Capsaicin, which desensitizes pain receptors.
- **Uses**: Applied topically in creams or patches to relieve nerve, muscle, and joint pain. Derived from chili peppers.

Digestive Disorders: Conditions such as irritable bowel syndrome (IBS) and acid reflux may benefit from dietary changes (e.g., elimination diets, probiotics), stress management techniques, and herbal remedies like **peppermint or ginger**. Also consider:

Chamomile:

- **Benefits**: Calms digestive spasms, reduces inflammation in the digestive tract, and promotes relaxation. It is often used to relieve indigestion and bloating.
- **Forms**: Chamomile tea is a popular form, but it can also be found in capsules or as an essential oil (for external use).

Fennel:

- **Benefits**: Relieves bloating, gas, and abdominal cramps. Fennel seeds can help stimulate digestion and reduce inflammation in the digestive tract.
- **Forms**: Fennel tea, fennel seeds (chewed or added to cooking), or fennel seed capsules.

Licorice Root:

- **Benefits**: Soothes the lining of the stomach and intestines, reduces inflammation, and supports overall digestive health. It may help with symptoms of acid reflux and indigestion.
- **Forms**: Licorice root tea, licorice root extract, or licorice root capsules (DGL - deglycyrrhizinated licorice).

Turmeric:

- **Benefits**: Has anti-inflammatory properties that can help reduce inflammation in the digestive tract. Turmeric supports liver function and bile production, aiding digestion.
- **Forms**: Turmeric can be used in cooking (as a spice), as a tea, or taken in supplement form (often combined with black pepper for better absorption).

Cardiovascular Health: Holistic approaches including dietary changes (e.g., Mediterranean diet), regular exercise, stress reduction techniques (e.g., Stretch techniques, meditation), and supplementation (e.g., omega-3 fatty acids) can support heart health and manage conditions like hypertension and high cholesterol.

Hawthorn:

- **Benefits**: Supports heart health by dilating blood vessels, improving circulation, and strengthening heart muscles. It may help manage high blood pressure, angina, and congestive heart failure.

- **Forms**: Hawthorn berries can be used to make tea, extracts, or capsules.

Garlic:

- **Benefits**: Has cardiovascular benefits including lowering blood pressure, reducing cholesterol levels, and improving circulation. Garlic also has anti-inflammatory and antioxidant properties.
- **Forms**: Fresh garlic (used in cooking), garlic supplements (powder, capsules, or aged garlic extract).

Ginger:

- **Benefits**: Helps lower blood pressure, reduce cholesterol levels, and improve blood circulation. Ginger also has anti-inflammatory properties that support cardiovascular health.
- **Forms**: Fresh ginger (used in cooking or tea), ginger capsules, or ginger extract.

Turmeric:

- **Benefits**: Contains curcumin, which has anti-inflammatory and antioxidant properties. Turmeric supports cardiovascular health by improving blood vessel function, reducing plaque buildup, and lowering cholesterol levels.
- **Forms**: Turmeric can be used in cooking (as a spice), as a tea, or taken in supplement form (often combined with black pepper for better absorption).

Ginkgo Biloba:

- **Benefits**: Improves circulation, enhances blood flow to the brain and extremities, and has antioxidant properties that protect blood vessels. It may help manage symptoms of peripheral artery disease (PAD).
- **Forms**: Ginkgo biloba extract is commonly used in capsules or tablets.

Cayenne Pepper:

- **Benefits**: Contains capsaicin, which helps improve circulation, reduce blood pressure, and support heart health. Cayenne pepper may also aid in digestion and metabolism.

- **Forms**: Cayenne pepper can be used as a spice in cooking, added to teas, or taken in capsule form.

Autoimmune Disorders: Holistic approaches focusing on diet (e.g., anti-inflammatory diets), stress reduction, supplementation (e.g., vitamin D, omega-3), and mind-body therapies (e.g., tai chi, acupuncture) may help manage symptoms of autoimmune conditions such as rheumatoid arthritis, lupus, and multiple sclerosis.

Respiratory Conditions: Asthma and chronic obstructive pulmonary disease (COPD) may benefit from holistic approaches such as breathing exercises (e.g., pranayama) and maintaining a healthy lifestyle to support lung function.

Eucalyptus:

- **Benefits**: Acts as an expectorant, helping to loosen phlegm and ease congestion. Eucalyptus also has anti-inflammatory and antimicrobial properties.
- **Forms**: Eucalyptus essential oil (for inhalation or chest rubs), dried leaves for tea, or eucalyptus extracts.

Peppermint:

- **Benefits**: Contains menthol, which helps relax the muscles of the respiratory tract and promote easier breathing. Peppermint also has anti-inflammatory properties.
- **Forms**: Peppermint tea, essential oil (for inhalation), or dried leaves for tea.

Ginger:

- **Benefits**: Has anti-inflammatory properties that can help soothe irritated airways and reduce inflammation in conditions like asthma and bronchitis.
- **Forms**: Fresh ginger root (used in cooking or tea), ginger capsules, or ginger extract.

Licorice Root:

- **Benefits**: Soothes inflammation in the respiratory tract and helps loosen mucus. It has expectorant properties that can aid in clearing the airways.

- **Forms**: Licorice root tea, licorice root extract, or licorice root capsules (DGL - deglycyrrhizinated licorice).

Thyme:

- **Benefits**: Contains compounds like thymol that have antimicrobial and expectorant properties. Thyme can help relieve coughs and support respiratory health.
- **Forms**: Thyme tea (from dried leaves), thyme essential oil (for inhalation), or thyme extracts.

Oregano:

- **Benefits**: Has antimicrobial properties that can help fight respiratory infections. Oregano also has antioxidant and anti-inflammatory effects.
- **Forms**: Oregano oil (for inhalation or diluted for topical use), dried oregano leaves for tea, or oregano extracts.

Skin Conditions: Holistic approaches including dietary changes (e.g., elimination of inflammatory foods), stress reduction techniques, and topical herbal treatments (e.g., calendula for eczema) can support skin health and manage conditions like eczema and acne.

Calendula:

- **Benefits**: Has anti-inflammatory, antimicrobial, and wound-healing properties. Calendula is used to soothe irritated skin, promote healing of wounds and burns, and reduce inflammation.
- **Forms**: Calendula cream or ointment, infused oils, or dried flowers for teas and washes.

Chamomile:

- **Benefits**: Calms inflamed skin and helps reduce itching and irritation. Chamomile has anti-inflammatory, antimicrobial, and antioxidant properties.
- **Forms**: Chamomile tea (applied topically or used as a compress), chamomile essential oil (diluted for skin application), or chamomile creams.

Aloe Vera:

- **Benefits**: Known for its soothing and moisturizing properties. Aloe vera helps reduce inflammation, promote healing of minor burns and wounds, and moisturize dry skin.
- **Forms**: Fresh aloe vera gel (directly from the plant), aloe vera creams or lotions, or aloe vera juice (used internally and externally).

Lavender:

- **Benefits**: Has anti-inflammatory, antimicrobial, and calming properties. Lavender is used to soothe irritated skin, reduce redness, and promote relaxation.
- **Forms**: Lavender essential oil (diluted for skin application), lavender-infused oils, or dried lavender flowers for baths and compresses.

Tea Tree Oil:

- **Benefits**: Antimicrobial and anti-inflammatory properties make tea tree oil effective for treating acne, fungal infections (like athlete's foot), and other skin conditions.

- **Forms**: Tea tree essential oil (diluted for skin application), tea tree creams or ointments, or tea tree soap.

Chapter 10: Decreasing the sugar

Processed sugar is considered detrimental to health for several reasons, primarily due to its impact on various bodily functions and systems. Processed sugar, such as sucrose and high-fructose corn syrup, provides "empty" calories, meaning it lacks essential nutrients like vitamins, minerals, and fiber. Consuming too much sugar can contribute to weight gain and obesity. Sugary foods and beverages cause rapid spikes in blood sugar levels, leading to a surge in insulin production by the pancreas. Over time, this can contribute to insulin resistance, a precursor to type 2 diabetes. Excessive sugar intake has been linked to an increased risk of chronic diseases such as type 2 diabetes, heart disease, and fatty liver disease. It can also exacerbate inflammation in the body, which is associated with various health problems.

Sugar promotes the growth of harmful bacteria in the mouth, leading to dental cavities and gum disease. This effect is exacerbated when sugary foods are consumed frequently or remain in contact with teeth for prolonged periods. High sugar intake can disrupt hormonal balance and metabolism, leading to increased fat accumulation, especially around the abdomen (visceral fat), which is a risk factor for metabolic syndrome.

Sugar can trigger the brain's reward system, leading to cravings and potentially addictive behaviors similar to those associated with drugs. Foods high in processed sugar often displace healthier, nutrient-dense foods in the diet. This can lead to deficiencies in essential nutrients necessary for overall health and well-being.

Be mindful of hidden sugars in processed foods, condiments, and beverages. Ingredients like sucrose, high-fructose corn syrup, and syrups indicate added sugars. Opt for whole fruits and vegetables, whole grains, lean proteins, and healthy fats instead of sugary snacks and desserts.
Avoid sugary sodas, energy drinks, and sweetened beverages. Opt for water, herbal teas, or unsweetened alternatives.

Prepare meals and snacks at home to control ingredients and reduce added sugars in your diet. Enjoy sugary treats occasionally and in moderation, focusing on overall balanced nutrition. By reducing processed sugar intake and focusing on whole, nutrient-dense foods, individuals can support better overall health and reduce the risk of chronic diseases associated with excessive sugar consumption.

Meals prepared with natural sugars

Meals prepared with natural sugars can be a delicious way to enjoy sweet flavors while incorporating nutrient-rich ingredients. Here are some examples of meals that use natural sugars:

1. **Fruit Salad**: Combine a variety of fresh fruits such as berries, melons, citrus fruits, and grapes. Natural sugars in fruits like strawberries, oranges, and grapes provide sweetness without added sugars.
2. **Oatmeal with Fruit**: Cook oats in water or milk and top with sliced bananas, berries, or diced apples. Sprinkle it with cinnamon for added flavor.

3. **Smoothie Bowl**: Blend together frozen bananas, berries, spinach, and a splash of almond milk for a thick, creamy smoothie base. Top with granola, coconut flakes, and fresh fruit for sweetness.

4. **Roasted Vegetables**: Roast sweet vegetables such as sweet potatoes, carrots, and beets with a drizzle of olive oil and a sprinkle of cinnamon or herbs. The natural sugars in the vegetables caramelize during roasting, enhancing their sweetness.

5. **Stir-Fry with Teriyaki Sauce**: Stir-fry vegetables, tofu, or chicken with a homemade teriyaki sauce made from soy sauce, honey or maple syrup, garlic, and ginger. The natural sugars in the honey or maple syrup add a touch of sweetness to the savory dish.

6. **Baked Apples**: Core apples and fill with a mixture of oats, nuts, cinnamon, and a drizzle of honey or maple syrup. Bake until tender for a warm and comforting dessert or snack.

7. **Yogurt Parfait**: Layer Greek yogurt with fresh berries, sliced bananas, and a sprinkle of nuts or granola. Drizzle with a little honey or maple syrup for added sweetness.

8. **Chia Seed Pudding**: Mix chia seeds with almond milk and sweeten with mashed ripe bananas or a touch of maple syrup. Let it sit overnight to thicken, then top with fresh fruit and nuts.

9. **Baked Acorn Squash**: Cut acorn squash in half, remove seeds, and roast with a drizzle of olive oil and a sprinkle of brown sugar or honey until tender. Serve as a side dish or stuffed with a savory filling.

10. **Homemade Granola Bars**: Make your own granola bars using rolled oats, nuts, seeds, dried fruit, and a binder like mashed dates or applesauce. Avoiding refined sugars, you can sweeten them naturally with honey or maple syrup.

These meals showcase the versatility of natural sugars from fruits, vegetables, and minimally processed sweeteners like honey and maple syrup. They provide a balance of flavors and nutrients, making them a healthy choice for satisfying your sweet cravings.

Chapter 11: Vitamins and Minerals

Vitamins and minerals are essential nutrients that play crucial roles in maintaining overall health and supporting various bodily functions. They act as coenzymes, which are necessary for many enzymatic reactions within cells. These reactions are vital for processes such as energy production, metabolism, and cellular repair. Many vitamins and minerals, such as vitamins A, C, D, E, and zinc, play key roles in supporting immune function. They help regulate immune responses, promote the production of immune cells, and protect against infections.

Minerals like calcium, phosphorus, magnesium, and vitamin D are essential for maintaining strong and healthy bones. They contribute to bone structure, density, and strength, helping to prevent conditions like osteoporosis. B vitamins (e.g., B1, B6, and B12) are crucial for nerve function and the synthesis of neurotransmitters. Minerals like magnesium and potassium also support nerve transmission and muscle function.

Many B vitamins, such as thiamine (B1), riboflavin (B2), niacin (B3), pantothenic acid (B5), and biotin (B7), play roles in converting food into energy through their involvement in carbohydrate, fat, and protein metabolism. Vitamins C and E, along with minerals like selenium and zinc, act as antioxidants that help neutralize harmful free radicals in the body. This protects cells from oxidative stress and damage.

Vitamin K is essential for proper blood clotting. It helps produce proteins that are necessary for the clotting process, which is crucial for wound healing and preventing excessive bleeding. Vitamins A, C, and E, as well as minerals like zinc and selenium, support healthy vision and skin by promoting tissue growth and repair, protecting against UV damage, and maintaining moisture and elasticity. Certain vitamins and minerals, including B vitamins (e.g., folate, B12) and magnesium, play roles in neurotransmitter synthesis and regulation. They are important for mood stability and mental health.

Obtaining Vitamins and Minerals

- **Diet**: The best way to obtain vitamins and minerals is through a balanced diet that includes a variety of nutrient-rich foods such as fruits, vegetables, whole grains, lean proteins, and dairy or dairy alternatives.
- **Supplements**: In some cases, dietary supplements may be recommended to ensure adequate intake of specific vitamins and minerals, especially for individuals with nutrient deficiencies or specific health conditions. However, supplements should be used under the guidance of a healthcare provider.

By ensuring an adequate intake of vitamins and minerals through a balanced diet and, when necessary, supplements, individuals can support overall health, optimize bodily functions, and reduce the risk of nutrient deficiencies and related health problems.

Mineral Deficiency

Mineral deficiency occurs when the body does not obtain or absorb enough of a specific mineral necessary for optimal health and function. Minerals play essential roles in various bodily processes, and deficiencies can lead to a range of health problems. Iron is critical for making hemoglobin, which carries oxygen in the blood. Iron deficiency can lead to anemia, characterized by fatigue, weakness, pale skin, and shortness of breath. It can also affect cognitive function and immune response.

Calcium is essential for bone health and muscle function. A deficiency can lead to osteoporosis (weakening of bones), muscle cramps, and an increased risk of fractures. In severe cases, it may affect heart function. Magnesium is involved in hundreds of enzymatic reactions in the body, including energy production and muscle function. Deficiency can lead to muscle cramps, fatigue, irregular heartbeat, and mood disturbances.

Zinc is important for immune function, wound healing, and DNA synthesis. Deficiency can lead to impaired immune response, delayed wound healing, hair loss, and skin problems. Iodine is crucial for thyroid function and the production of thyroid hormones. Deficiency can lead to thyroid disorders, such as goiter (enlargement of the thyroid gland) and hypothyroidism (underactive thyroid). Selenium is an antioxidant that plays a role in thyroid function and immune response. Deficiency may impair thyroid function, weaken immune defenses, and increase the risk of certain cancers. Potassium is important for nerve transmission, muscle function, and maintaining electrolyte balance. Deficiency can cause muscle weakness, cramps, irregular heartbeat, and in severe cases, paralysis.

Causes of Mineral Deficiency:

- **Inadequate Intake**: Not consuming enough foods rich in specific minerals.
- **Poor Absorption**: Conditions that affect the absorption of minerals from the digestive tract, such as celiac disease or inflammatory bowel diseases.
- **Increased Needs**: During pregnancy, lactation, growth periods, or due to certain medical conditions.
- **Medications**: Some medications can interfere with mineral absorption or increase excretion.

Prevention and Treatment:

- **Balanced Diet**: Eating a variety of nutrient-dense foods, including fruits, vegetables, whole grains, lean proteins, and dairy or dairy alternatives rich in minerals.
- **Supplementation**: In cases of deficiency, supplements may be recommended under medical supervision to restore optimal levels.
- **Medical Evaluation**: If symptoms suggest a mineral deficiency, a healthcare provider can conduct tests to diagnose the deficiency and recommend appropriate treatment.

Addressing mineral deficiencies promptly is important for maintaining overall health and preventing long-term complications. It's essential to consult with a healthcare provider for proper diagnosis and treatment of any suspected mineral deficiency.

The following questions are to review your knowledge and understanding on the importance of minerals for the body.

What do you understand about the importance of minerals in the body?

Have you ever experienced symptoms that could be related to a mineral deficiency?

How do you ensure you get enough minerals in your diet?

Are there any specific minerals you are aware of and their roles in health?

Do you think mineral deficiencies are common in our society today? Why or why not?

Have you ever taken supplements for mineral deficiencies? How did they affect you?

What are some common signs or symptoms of mineral deficiencies that people should be aware of?

How can lifestyle choices like diet and exercise impact mineral levels in the body?

What are some factors that might contribute to mineral deficiencies in individuals?

How important do you think it is to regularly monitor mineral levels in the body?

Chapter 12: Creating a Holistic Lifestyle

Incorporating holistic practices into daily life involves integrating various aspects of health and wellness to achieve overall well-being. Here are some key tips for adopting and maintaining a holistic lifestyle:

1. **Mindful Awareness**: Start by becoming aware of your current habits and how they impact your overall health. Mindfulness helps you recognize areas where you can make positive changes.
2. **Balanced Nutrition**: Focus on consuming a balanced diet rich in whole foods, including fruits, vegetables, whole grains, lean proteins, and healthy fats. Minimize processed foods and sugars.
3. **Regular Physical Activity**: Incorporate regular exercise into your routine, including cardio, strength training, and flexibility exercises like yoga or tai chi. Find activities you enjoy to stay motivated.
4. **Stress Management**: Practice stress-reducing techniques such as meditation, deep breathing exercises, yoga, or spending time in nature. These practices help alleviate stress and promote mental clarity.

5. **Quality Sleep**: Prioritize sleep by establishing a consistent sleep schedule, creating a relaxing bedtime routine, and ensuring your sleep environment is conducive to restful sleep.
6. **Hydration**: Drink plenty of water throughout the day to stay hydrated and support bodily functions. Herbal teas and infused water can also provide hydration and additional health benefits.
7. **Social Connections**: Foster meaningful relationships and social connections with friends, family, and community. Strong social support can contribute to emotional well-being.
8. **Holistic Therapies**: Explore complementary therapies such as acupuncture, massage therapy, chiropractic care, or aromatherapy to support overall health and address specific health concerns.
9. **Self-Care Practices**: Dedicate time for self-care activities that nourish your mind, body, and spirit. This may include hobbies, relaxation techniques, or creative outlets.
10. **Goal Setting**: Set realistic and achievable health goals that align with your values and priorities. Break larger goals into smaller, manageable steps to track progress and stay motivated.

11. **Overcoming Challenges**: Identify common obstacles such as time constraints, stress, or lack of motivation, and develop strategies to overcome them. Seek support from others or professional guidance if needed.

12. **Long-Term Sustainability**: Focus on building sustainable habits rather than quick fixes. Embrace gradual changes and be patient with yourself as you adapt to a holistic lifestyle over time.

By incorporating these tips into daily life, individuals can cultivate a holistic approach to health that addresses physical, mental, emotional, and spiritual well-being, promoting long-term health and vitality.

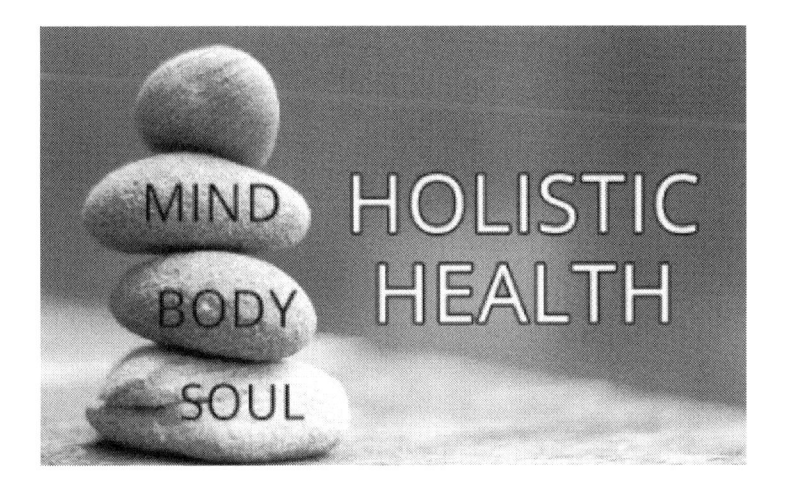

Achieving Your Best Health Holistically

Conclusion

Achieving your best health holistically involves integrating various aspects of wellness to nurture not just the body, but also the mind and spirit. By adopting a holistic approach, individuals can optimize their overall well-being and vitality in a sustainable manner. Here's a conclusion on the topic:

Holistic health emphasizes the interconnectedness of physical, mental, emotional, and spiritual aspects of our lives. It encourages us to take a comprehensive view of health, recognizing that factors like nutrition, exercise, sleep, stress management, and social connections all play pivotal roles in our well-being. By prioritizing whole foods, regular physical activity, adequate rest, and mindfulness practices, we support the body's natural ability to heal and thrive.

Moreover, holistic health empowers individuals to address the root causes of health issues rather than merely treating symptoms. It encourages preventive measures, such as maintaining a balanced diet rich in nutrients, managing stress effectively, and fostering supportive relationships. By embracing these principles, we not only enhance our physical health but also cultivate resilience, emotional stability, and a deeper sense of purpose in life.

In essence, achieving optimal health holistically is a journey that requires dedication, mindfulness, and a commitment to self-care. It's about making informed choices that nourish the body, mind, and spirit, ultimately leading to a more vibrant and fulfilling life. By embracing holistic practices, we pave the way for sustained health and well-being, empowering ourselves to live our best lives possible.

Resources for Further Reading

Here are some recommended resources for further reading on holistic health and achieving optimal well-being:

1. Books:
    - *The Complete Guide to Holistic Health* by David Hoffmann
    - *Mind Over Medicine: Scientific Proof That You Can Heal Yourself* by Lissa Rankin, MD
    - *The Holistic Health Handbook: A Tool for Attaining Wholeness of Body, Mind, and Spirit* by Berkeley Holistic Health Center
2. Websites and Online Resources:
    - National Center for Complementary and Integrative Health (NCCIH): Offers evidence-based information on complementary health approaches.
        - Website: https://www.nccih.nih.gov/
    - Holistic Health Tools: Provides articles and resources on holistic health practices and approaches.

- Website: https://www.holistichealthtools.com/
  - American Holistic Health Association (AHHA): Offers resources, articles, and directories for finding holistic practitioners.
    - Website: https://ahha.org/
  - Mindful: Offers articles and resources on mindfulness, meditation, and holistic living.
    - Website: https://www.mindful.org/
  - Top 10 Home Remedies

3. Journals and Publications:
   - *Journal of Alternative and Complementary Medicine*: Publishes research on integrative, holistic, and complementary approaches to health.
   - *Explore: The Journal of Science and Healing*: Focuses on holistic health and healing practices.
   - *Alternative Therapies in Health and Medicine*: Covers integrative approaches to health and wellness.

4. Podcasts and Online Courses:

- The Mindful Kind Podcast: Hosted by Rachael Kable, focusing on mindfulness and holistic well-being.
    - Website: https://www.rachaelkable.com/podcast
- Coursera: Offers online courses on holistic health, mindfulness, nutrition, and more from universities and institutions worldwide.
    - Website: https://www.coursera.org/
- Health Talk with Lisa
    - Health Talk with Dr. Lisa | WONIRadio
    - Home | The Holistic Balanced Life Center (balancedcare-aholisticlife.com)

These resources provide a wealth of information and insights into holistic health practices, mindfulness, nutrition, and integrative approaches to wellness. Whether you're looking for books to deepen your understanding, reputable websites for articles and tools, or educational platforms for courses, these resources can support your journey towards achieving optimal health holistically.

Quick and healthy meal recommendations

Here are some ideas for quick and healthy meals that you can prepare:

1. **Grilled Chicken Salad**: Grilled chicken breast served over mixed greens with cherry tomatoes, cucumber slices, and a light vinaigrette dressing.
2. **Stir-Fry with Vegetables**: Sautéed mixed vegetables (bell peppers, broccoli, carrots) with tofu or shrimp, seasoned with soy sauce and garlic, served over brown rice or quinoa.
3. **Avocado Toast**: Whole grain toast topped with mashed avocado, sliced tomatoes, a sprinkle of feta cheese, and a drizzle of olive oil.
4. **Vegetable Omelet**: Whisked eggs cooked with spinach, mushrooms, and bell peppers, folded over and served with a side of whole grain toast.
5. **Greek Yogurt Parfait**: Greek yogurt layered with fresh berries, nuts or granola, and a drizzle of honey or maple syrup.
6. **Quinoa Salad**: Cooked quinoa mixed with diced cucumbers, cherry tomatoes, black beans, corn, and a lime-cilantro dressing.

7. **Salmon with Steamed Vegetables**: Baked or grilled salmon fillet served with steamed broccoli, carrots, and a side of wild rice.

8. **Black Bean Tacos**: Whole grain tortillas filled with black beans, shredded lettuce, diced tomatoes, avocado slices, and a squeeze of lime.

9. **Caprese Sandwich**: Whole grain bread sandwiched with fresh mozzarella cheese, sliced tomatoes, basil leaves, and a drizzle of balsamic glaze.

10. **Mango Chicken Wraps**: Whole wheat tortillas filled with grilled chicken breast, mixed greens, sliced mango, and a light yogurt or avocado dressing.

These meals are quick to prepare, balanced in nutrients, and provide a variety of flavors and textures to keep your meals interesting and satisfying. Adjust ingredients based on your preferences and dietary needs for optimal health and enjoyment.

Reference Page

Books

- Hoffmann, David. *The Complete Guide to Holistic Health*. Healing Arts Press, 2002.
- Rankin, Lissa. *Mind Over Medicine: Scientific Proof That You Can Heal Yourself*. Hay House, 2013.
- Berkeley Holistic Health Center. *The Holistic Health Handbook: A Tool for Attaining Wholeness of Body, Mind, and Spirit*. Random House, 2005.
- Bible, NIV. (2011). *Holy Bible: New International Version*. Zondervan.

Websites and Online Resources

- National Center for Complementary and Integrative Health (NCCIH). "National Institutes of Health". https://www.nccih.nih.gov/
- Holistic Health Tools. "Holistic Health Tools". https://www.holistichealthtools.com/

- American Holistic Health Association (AHHA). "AHHA". https://ahha.org/

- Mindful. "Mindful". https://www.mindful.org/

Journals and Publications

- Journal of Alternative and Complementary Medicine. Mary Ann Liebert, Inc., https://home.liebertpub.com/publications/journal-of-alternative-and-complementary-medicine/51

- Explore: The Journal of Science and Healing. Elsevier, https://www.journals.elsevier.com/explore-the-journal-of-science-and-healing/

- Alternative Therapies in Health and Medicine. InnoVision Health Media, https://www.alternative-therapies.com/

This page was intentionally left blank

Made in the USA
Columbia, SC
13 August 2024